Asian vegan cookbook

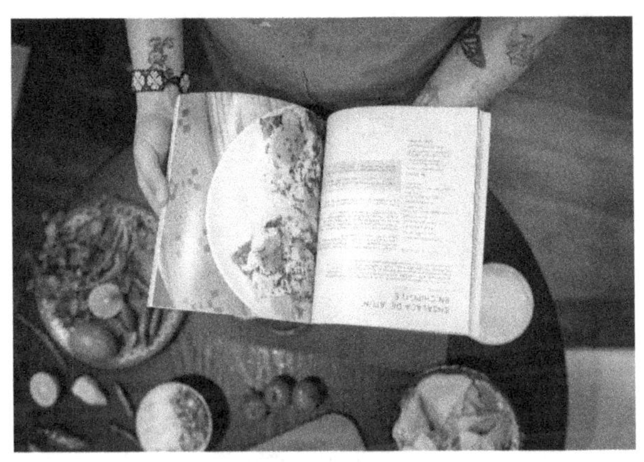

Explore Flavorful Plant-Based Delights from the East

Violet M. Schulze

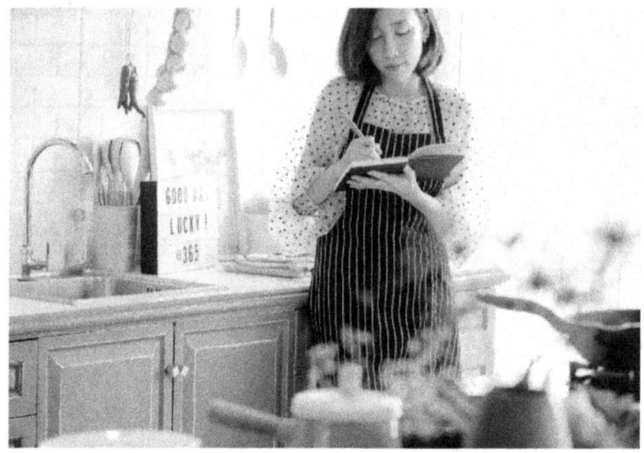
GOOD
LUCKY
365

Table of contents

Introduction to Asian Vegan Cuisine

Rich culinary traditions and plant-based products that satisfy the palate and feed the body are combined to create Asian vegan food. Asian vegan food gives both vegans and non-vegans a fascinating culinary experience with its rich diversity of tastes, textures, and spices.

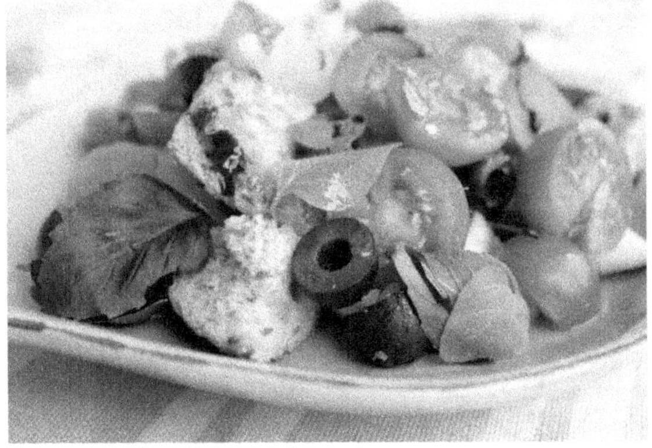

Asian vegan food has become more and more popular in recent years as people look for more sustainable and healthful food alternatives. Through the use of plant-based ingredients and cooking methods from traditional Asian cuisine, chefs have elevated everyday meals into inventive, plant-based masterpieces

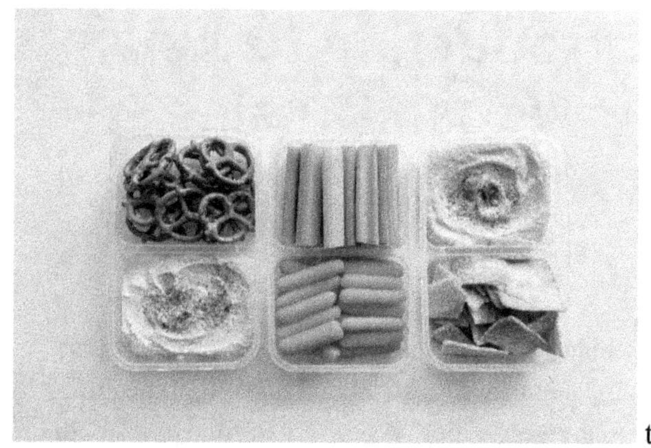 that
honor the abundance of nature.

A wide variety of fresh fruits, veggies, grains, and legumes are the foundation of Asian vegan cooking. Asian vegan cuisines highlight the diversity and availability of plant-based foods available, from the creamy richness of coconut-based curries to the crisp bite of stir-fried bok cabbage.

Asian vegan cooking is known for emphasizing strong tastes and fragrant spices. Herbs with strong flavor, such as garlic and chili peppers, give food a scorching rush that awakens the palate. Fragrant herbs, such as lemongrass, ginger, and cilantro, provide meals depth and complexity.

Asian vegan food provides a wide range of culinary pleasures, from the delicious comfort of hot bowls of vegan ramen to the delicate balance of tastes in sushi rolls loaded with crisp vegetables. Every meal, whether it's savoring the delicious aromas of Indian dal or a

steaming bow
invention, in

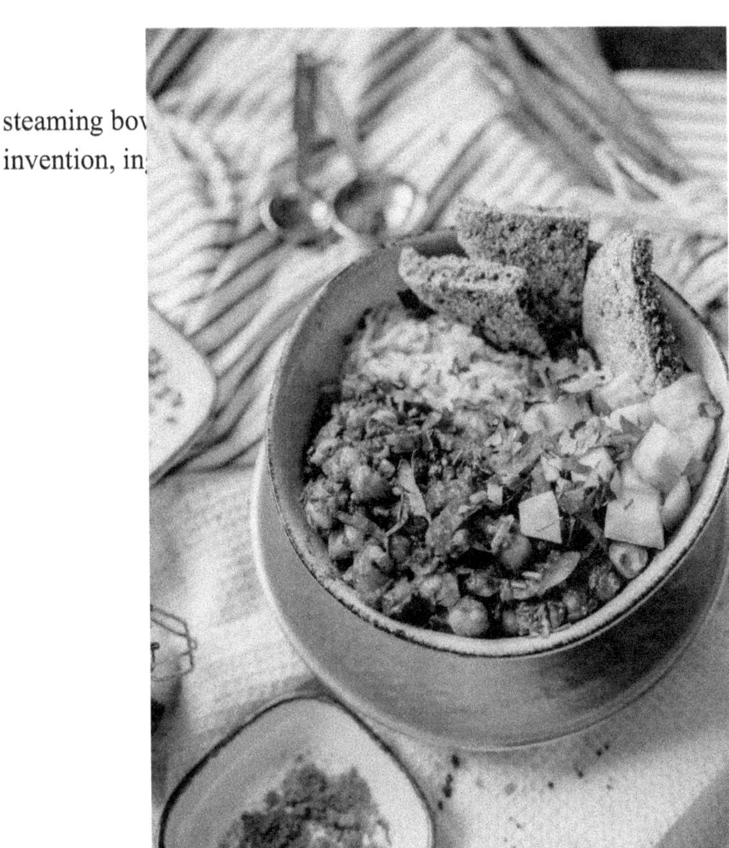

Essential Ingredients in Asian Vegan Cooking

- **Tofu and Tempeh:** Commonly used in Asian cuisine, tofu, which is derived from soybeans, and tempeh, which is prepared from fermented soybeans, are adaptable plant-based protein sources. They provide food texture and richness by absorbing the tastes of sauces and marinades.

- **veggies:** The foundation of Asian vegan food is an extensive assortment of fresh veggies. Vegetables give meals vital nutrients, texture, and flavor. Examples of these include colorful bell peppers, carrots, and broccoli, as well as lush greens like spinach and bok choy.

- **Noodles and rice:** These two items are used in many Asian vegan recipes. These starches make a filling foundation for stir-fries, curries, and noodle bowls, whether they're served as chewy rice noodles, aromatic basmati rice, or steamed jasmine rice.

- **Coconut Milk and Cream:** Asian vegan curries, soups, and desserts benefit from the richness and creaminess that coconut milk and cream provide. They enhance savory and spicy foods with a delicate sweetness and depth of taste.

- **Herbs & Spices with Aromas:** Deep flavor and complexity may be achieved in Asian vegan recipes by including aromatic herbs and spices such as curry leaves, ginger, garlic, cilantro, turmeric, and lemongrass. They enhance food with strong tastes and enticing scents that entice the senses.

- **Soy Sauce and Tamari:** In Asian vegan cookery, soy sauce and tamari, a gluten-free substitute, are essential condiments. They improve the overall flavor of foods by contributing a salty, umami flavor to marinades, stir-fries, and dipping sauces.

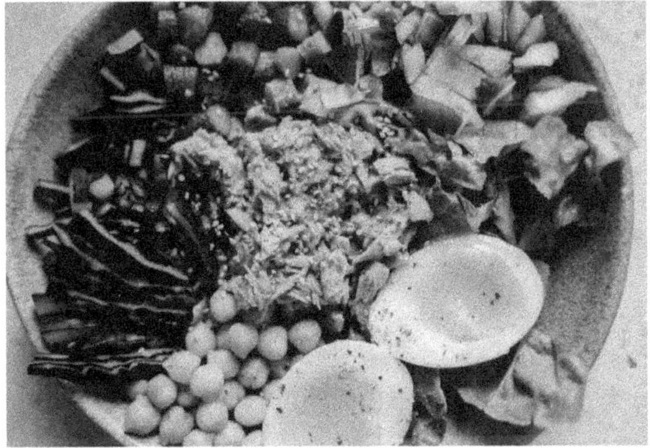

- **Seaweed and Nori:** These ingredients give Asian vegan cuisine a faintly aquatic taste. They frequently offer nutritious value and a subtle umami flavor to sushi rolls, salads, and soups.

- **Sesame Oil and Seeds:** In Asian vegan cookery, sesame oil and seeds are highly valued for their nutty flavor and scent. They impart a unique fl[...]ed, a[...].

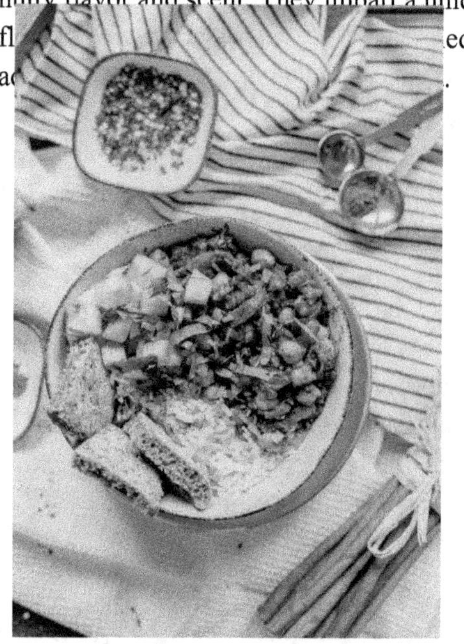

Appetizers and Starters

Vegetable Spring Rolls

Ingredients:

For the Spring Rolls:

- 12 spring roll wrappers (rice paper)
- 1 cup shredded lettuce
- 1 cup shredded cabbage
- 1 carrot, julienned
- 1 cucumber, julienned
- 1 bell pepper, thinly sliced
- 1 avocado, thinly sliced
- 1/2 cup fresh mint leaves
- 1/2 cup fresh cilantro leaves
- 1/2 cup fresh basil leaves

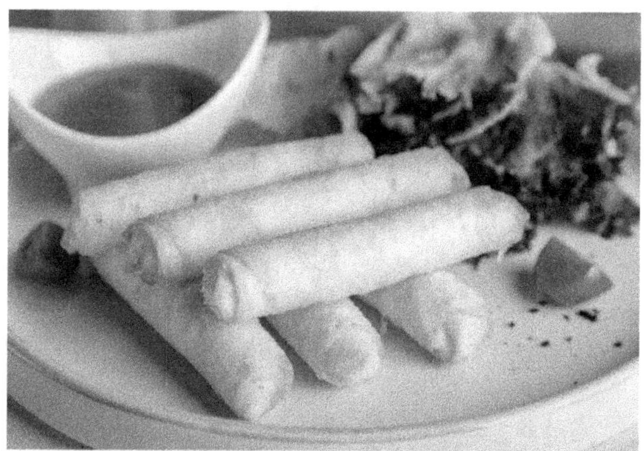

For the Dipping Sauce:

- 1/4 cup soy sauce or tamari
- 2 tablespoons rice vinegar
- 1 tablespoon maple syrup or coconut sugar
- 1 teaspoon sesame oil
- 1 teaspoon grated ginger
- 1 clove garlic, minced
- 1 tablespoon chopped green onions (optional)
- 1 teaspoon chili garlic sauce (optional)

Instructions:

- Wash, peel, and thinly slice all the veggies to prepare them.
- Pour some warm water into a small dish. One rice paper wrapper should be dipped into the water for five to ten seconds to make it malleable. It should be put on a fresh, moist kitchen towel.

- Leaving approximately 2 inches of room on each side, arrange a small quantity of shredded lettuce, cabbage, carrot, cucumber, bell pepper, avocado, mint, cilantro, and basil leaves in the middle of the rice paper wrapper.
- To create a spring roll, fold the bottom of the wrapper over the filling, tuck the edges in, and roll firmly. Proceed with the remaining wrappers and ingredients for the filling.
- In order to prepare the dipping sauce, thoroughly mix the soy sauce (or tamari), rice vinegar, maple syrup (or coconut sugar), sesame oil, grated ginger, minced garlic, chopped green onions (if desired), and chili garlic sauce (if applicable) in a small dish.
- Present the veggie spring rolls beside the accompanying dipping sauce.

Edamame Dumplings

Ingredients:

For the Dumpling Filling:

- 1 cup shelled edamame (frozen or fresh)
- 1/2 cup firm tofu, drained and crumbled

- 2 cloves garlic, minced
- 1 tablespoon grated ginger
- 2 green onions, finely chopped
- 2 tablespoons soy sauce or tamari
- 1 tablespoon sesame oil
- 1 teaspoon rice vinegar
- Salt and pepper to taste

For the Dumpling Wrappers:

- 24 round dumpling wrappers (you can find these in the refrigerated section of most Asian grocery stores)

For the Dipping Sauce:

- 1/4 cup soy sauce or tamari
- 2 tablespoons rice vinegar
- 1 teaspoon sesame oil
- 1 teaspoon grated ginger
- 1 clove garlic, minced
- 1 tablespoon chopped green onions (optional)
- 1/2 teaspoon chili flakes (optional)

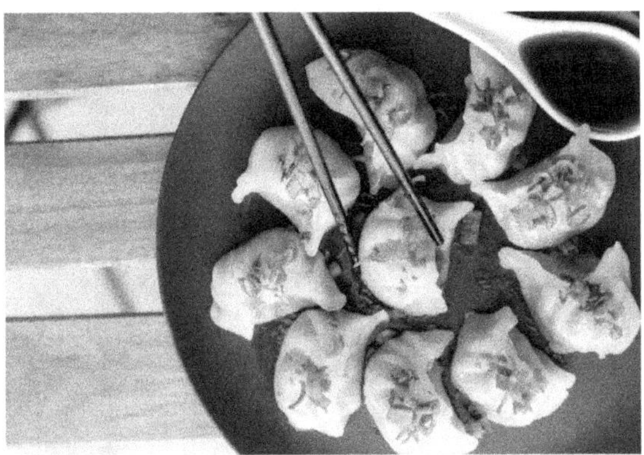

Instructions:

1. Boil the shelled edamame for three to five minutes, or until they are soft. After draining, leave to cool somewhat.
2. Cooked edamame, crumbled tofu, minced garlic, grated ginger, chopped green onions, sesame oil, rice vinegar, soy sauce (or tamari), salt, and pepper should all be combined in a food processor. Pulse the mixture until it's well mixed but has some chunks remaining.
3. Make a tiny indentation in the middle of each dumpling wrapper for the edamame filling.
4. With your fingertip, moisten the edges of the wrapper with water.
5. To form a half-moon, fold the dumpling wrapper in half over the filling. Make sure there are no air pockets by pressing the edges together to seal.
6. Holding the filled dumpling in one hand, make tiny pleats along the sealed edge by folding and pinching the edges together with your other

hand's thumb and index finger. Continue until you have pleated every dumpling.

7. To keep them from sticking, place the dumplings on a tray lined with parchment paper or a surface dusted with flour.
8. Cook the dumplings in batches in a large saucepan of boiling water for 4–5 minutes, or until the wrappers are cooked through and they float to the top.
9. Make the dipping sauce while the dumplings are cooking. Add the rice vinegar, sesame oil, grated ginger, minced garlic, chopped green onions (if used), soy sauce (or tamari), and chili flakes (if using) to a small bowl. Mix well to blend.
10. Present the heated edamame dumplings alongside the accompanying dipping sauce.

Vegan Sushi Rolls

Ingredients:

- 2 cups sushi rice
- 2 1/2 cups water
- 1/4 cup rice vinegar
- 2 tablespoons sugar
- 1 teaspoon salt

- Nori seaweed sheets
- Assorted vegetables (such as cucumber, avocado, carrot, bell pepper, and tofu)
- Soy sauce, for serving
- Pickled ginger, for serving
- Wasabi, for serving
- Bamboo sushi rolling mat

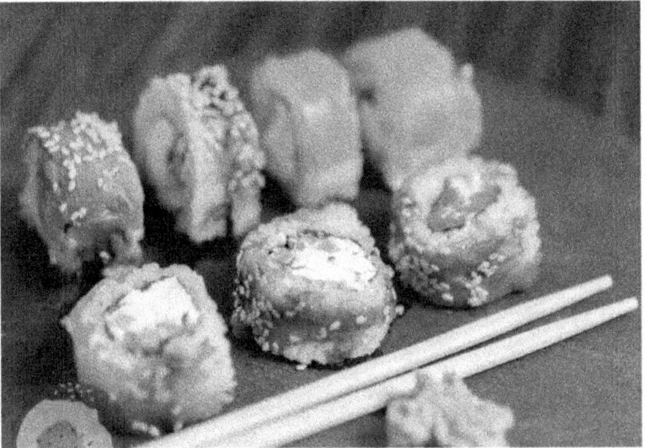

Instructions:

1. Till the water runs clear, rinse the sushi rice under cold water. Make sure to drain properly.
2. Rinse the sushi rice and add water to a medium pot. After bringing the rice to a boil, lower the heat to a simmer, cover, and cook for 18 to 20 minutes, or until the rice is soft and the water has been absorbed.
3. Mix the sugar, salt, and rice vinegar in a small bowl until the ingredients are dissolved.
4. Carefully incorporate the rice vinegar mixture into the cooked rice after transferring it to a big bowl, taking care not to crush it. Allow rice to reach room temperature.

5. Cut the tofu and veggies of your choosing into thin strips or julienne.
6. Arrange a nori seaweed sheet, shiny side down, on a sushi rolling mat made of bamboo.
7. Using moist hands, uniformly cover the nori seaweed with a thin coating of sushi rice, allowing about 1 inch of room at the top border.
8. Place the tofu and your preferred veggies in a line across the middle of the rice.
9. Tuck the contents firmly within the sushi by carefully rolling it away from you using the bamboo mat. To seal the roll, gently push down.
10. Proceed with the other components in the same manner.
11. After the sushi rolls are put together, cut each one into bite-sized pieces using a sharp knife.
12. Present the vegan sushi rolls alongside wasabi, pickled ginger, and soy sauce.
13. Savor your handmade vegan sushi rolls as a tasty and wholesome snack or dinner!

Thai Mango Salad

Ingredients:

- 2 ripe mangoes, peeled and sliced into thin strips
- 1 red bell pepper, thinly sliced
- 1/2 red onion, thinly sliced

- 1/4 cup fresh cilantro leaves, chopped
- 1/4 cup fresh mint leaves, chopped
- 1/4 cup roasted peanuts, chopped
- 2 tablespoons lime juice
- 1 tablespoon soy sauce or tamari
- 1 tablespoon maple syrup or brown sugar
- 1 tablespoon sesame oil
- 1 teaspoon grated ginger
- 1 garlic clove, minced
- Red chili flakes, to taste (optional)
- Salt, to taste

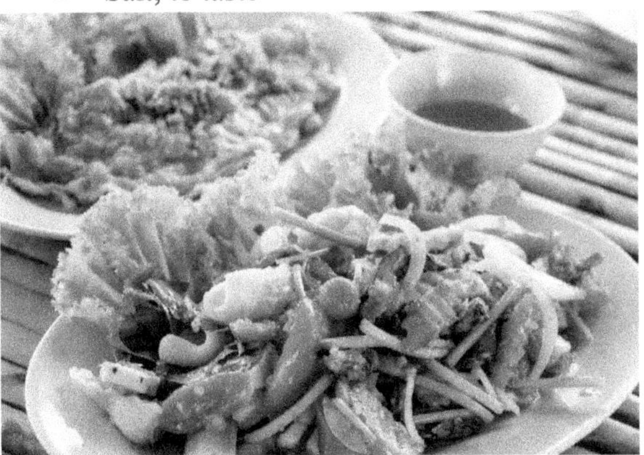

Instructions:

1. Mango slices, red bell pepper, red onion, cilantro, mint, and chopped peanuts should all be combined in a big dish.
2. Lime juice, soy sauce, maple syrup (or brown sugar), sesame oil, chopped garlic, grated ginger, red chili flakes (if used), and salt to taste should all be combined in a separate small dish.
3. After adding the dressing to the mango salad, gently toss to cover every component equally.

4. Give the salad ten to fifteen minutes to marinade
    so that the flavors may combine.
5. If preferred, top the chilled or room temperature
    Thai mango salad with more chopped peanuts
    and fresh herbs.
6. Savor this colorful and crisp Thai mango salad
    as an appetizer or a light dinner!

Noodle and Rice Dishes

Vegan Pad Thai

Ingredients:

- 8 ounces rice noodles
- 2 tablespoons soy sauce or tamari
- 2 tablespoons tamarind paste
- 2 tablespoons maple syrup or coconut sugar
- 1 tablespoon lime juice
- 2 tablespoons peanut or sesame oil
- 1 block (about 14 ounces) firm tofu, pressed and cubed
- 2 cloves garlic, minced
- 1 small onion, thinly sliced
- 1 cup shredded carrots
- 1 bell pepper, thinly sliced
- 1 cup bean sprouts
- 2 green onions, chopped
- 1/4 cup chopped peanuts (optional)
- Lime wedges, for serving
- Fresh cilantro, for garnish

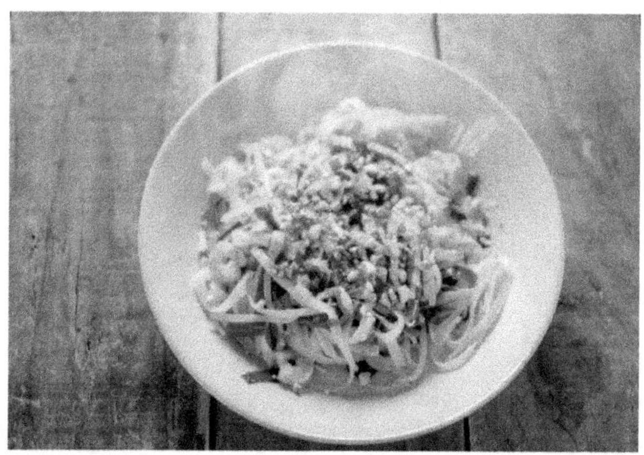

Instructions:

1. Cook the rice noodles until they are al dente, following the directions on the package. After draining, set away.
2. To prepare the sauce, combine the tamarind paste, lime juice, maple syrup (or coconut sugar), and soy sauce (or tamari) in a small bowl. Put aside.
3. Heat the sesame or peanut oil in a big wok or pan over medium-high heat. Add the cubed tofu and heat for 5 to 7 minutes, or until golden brown on both sides. Take out and put aside the tofu from the pan.
4. Add the onion slices and minced garlic to the same skillet. Stir-fry for two to three minutes, or until aromatic and beginning to soften.
5. Add sliced bell pepper and shredded carrots to skillet. Simmer for a further 3–4 minutes, or until the veggies are crisp-tender.

6. Put the cooked tofu back in the skillet. Add the bean sprouts and cooked rice noodles.
7. Cover the noodles and veggies in the pan with sauce. Mix everything thoroughly until thoroughly hot, which should take two to three minutes.
8. Take the pan off of the burner and, if desired, add some chopped peanuts and green onions as garnish.
9. Serve Pad Thai hot, with fresh cilantro and lime wedges as garnish.

Vegetable Fried Rice

Ingredients:

- 2 cups cooked rice, preferably chilled
- 2 tablespoons vegetable oil
- 1 onion, diced
- 2 cloves garlic, minced
- 1 cup mixed vegetables (such as peas, carrots, corn, and bell peppers)
- 2 tablespoons soy sauce or tamari
- 1 tablespoon sesame oil
- 2 green onions, chopped
- Salt and pepper to taste

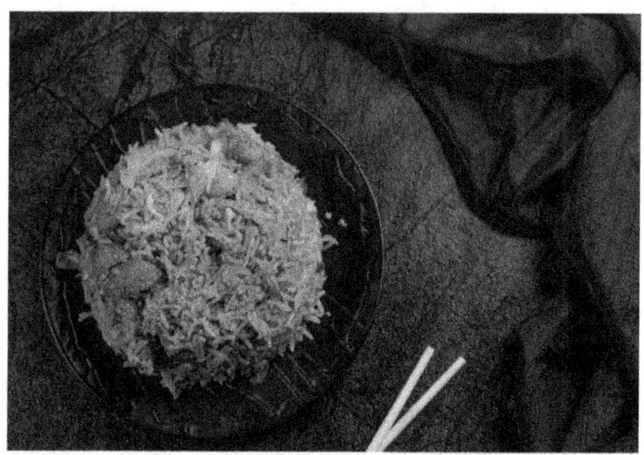

Instructions:

1. In a large skillet or wok, heat the vegetable oil over medium-high heat.
2. Add minced garlic and chopped onion to the skillet. Simmer the onion for 3–4 minutes, or until it is transparent.
3. Cook the mixed veggies in the pan for five to six minutes, or until they are soft.
4. When the rice is done, add it to the skillet and stir-fry it for two to three minutes.
5. Over the rice mixture, drizzle sesame oil and soy sauce (or tamari). Mix everything together.
6. Toss everything together in the skillet after adding the chopped green onions.
7. To taste, add salt and pepper for seasoning.
8. Serve hot vegetable fried rice as a filling main meal or side.

Japanese Ramen Soup

Note: Japanese ramen soup comes in a variety of forms. This is a simple recipe:

Ingredients:

- 4 cups vegetable broth
- 2 cloves garlic, minced
- 1 tablespoon grated ginger
- 2 tablespoons soy sauce or tamari
- 1 tablespoon miso paste
- 2 bundles of ramen noodles
- Toppings of your choice (such as sliced tofu, mushrooms, green onions, spinach, seaweed, and corn)

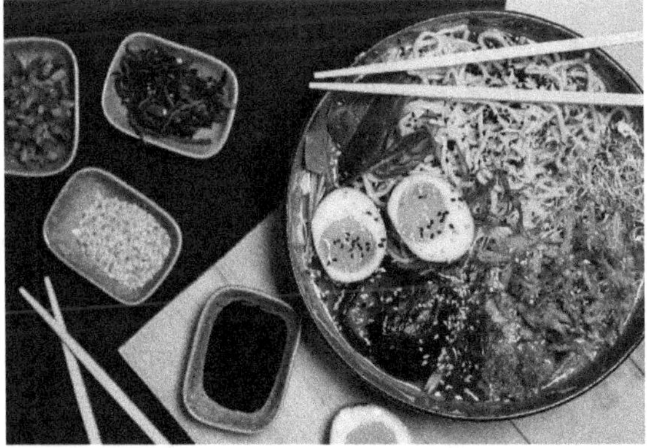

Instructions:

1. Heat a large saucepan over medium heat and add the veggie broth.

2. Toss in the miso paste, grated ginger, chopped garlic, and soy sauce (or tamari). To enable the flavors to mingle, stir everything together and simmer for 5 to 10 minutes.

3. Follow the directions on the package to prepare the ramen noodles. After draining, set away.

4. Choose your toppings and cut or slice them according to your preference.

5. Spoon cooked ramen noodles into dishes for serving. Spoon hot consommé over noodles.

6. Place garnishes over the ramen soup.

7. Enjoy your hot Japanese ramen soup!

Singapore Noodles

Ingredients:

- 8 ounces rice vermicelli noodles
- 2 tablespoons vegetable oil
- 1 onion, thinly sliced
- 2 cloves garlic, minced
- 1 red bell pepper, thinly sliced
- 1 carrot, julienned
- 1 cup sliced mushrooms
- 1 cup bean sprouts
- 2 green onions, chopped
- 2 tablespoons soy sauce or tamari
- 1 tablespoon curry powder
- 1 teaspoon turmeric powder

- Salt and pepper to taste

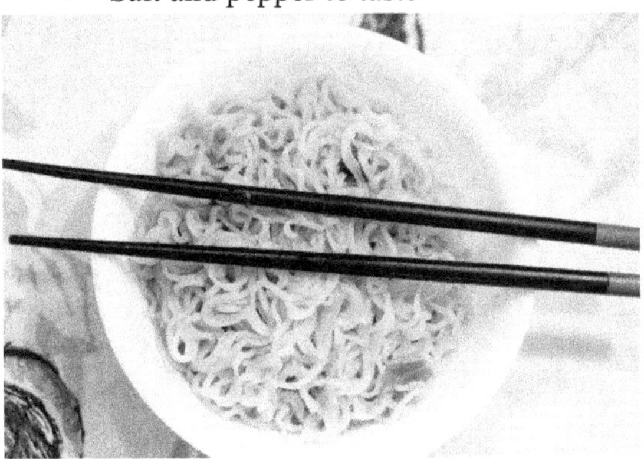

Instructions:

1. Follow the directions on the package to prepare the rice vermicelli noodles. After draining, set away.
2. In a large skillet or wok, heat the vegetable oil over medium-high heat.
3. Add minced garlic and thinly sliced onion to skillet. Simmer the onion for 3–4 minutes, or until it is transparent.
4. To the skillet, add the sliced mushrooms, julienned carrot, and red bell pepper. Stir-fry for 5 to 6 minutes, or until veggies are soft.
5. Stir the bean sprouts and cooked rice vermicelli noodles into the skillet. Mix everything together.
6. Combine the curry powder, turmeric powder, and soy sauce (or tamari) in a small bowl. Fill pan with noodle mixture; pour over.
7. Stir-fry noodles for 2 to 3 minutes, or until they are well warm and the sauce is uniformly covered.

8. To taste, add salt and pepper for seasoning.
9. Before serving, sprinkle chopped green onions over the Singapore noodles.
10. Serve hot for a filling and tasty supper. Have fun!

Tofu and Tempeh Creations

General Tso's Tofu

Ingredients:

For the Tofu:

- 1 block (about 14 ounces) firm tofu, pressed and cubed
- 1/4 cup cornstarch
- 2 tablespoons vegetable oil

For the Sauce:

- 1/4 cup soy sauce or tamari
- 2 tablespoons rice vinegar
- 2 tablespoons maple syrup or brown sugar
- 1 tablespoon hoisin sauce
- 1 tablespoon tomato paste
- 2 cloves garlic, minced
- 1 teaspoon grated ginger
- 1 teaspoon sesame oil
- 1 tablespoon cornstarch mixed with 2 tablespoons water (for thickening)

- Red pepper flakes or sriracha sauce, to taste (optional)
- Sliced green onions and sesame seeds, for garnish

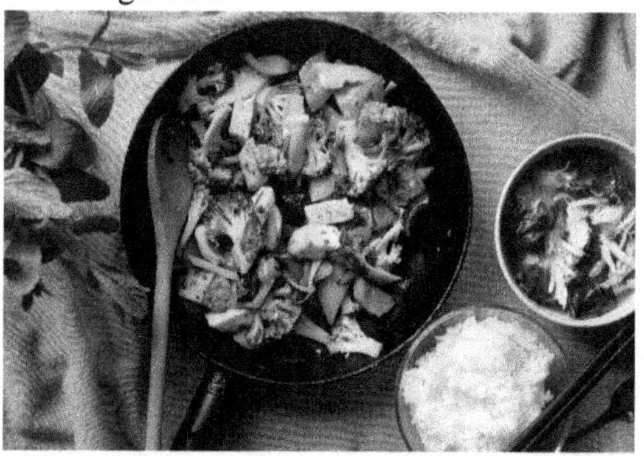

Instructions:

1. Coat the cubed tofu well with cornstarch.
2. In a big skillet, heat the vegetable oil over medium-high heat. After adding the tofu cubes, fry for 6 to 8 minutes, or until golden brown and crispy on both sides. Take out and put aside the tofu from the pan.
3. Add the rice vinegar, hoisin sauce, hoisin sauce, chopped garlic, grated ginger, soy sauce (or tamari), and sesame oil to the same skillet. Mix well to blend.
4. On medium heat, bring the sauce to a simmer. To thicken the sauce, stir in the cornstarch-water combination.
5. Return the cooked tofu to the skillet and stir to ensure that the sauce coats it evenly. Cook for a

further two to three minutes, or until well heated.

6. If desired, add more sriracha sauce or red pepper flakes to the seasoning.

7. Serve hot General Tso's tofu over cooked rice or noodles, topped with sesame seeds and sliced green onions.

Korean BBQ Tempeh

Ingredients:

- 1 block (about 8 ounces) tempeh, sliced into thin strips
- 1/4 cup soy sauce or tamari
- 2 tablespoons maple syrup or brown sugar
- 1 tablespoon sesame oil
- 2 cloves garlic, minced
- 1 teaspoon grated ginger
- 1 tablespoon rice vinegar
- 1 tablespoon gochujang (Korean chili paste)
- 1 tablespoon sesame seeds
- Sliced green onions, for garnish

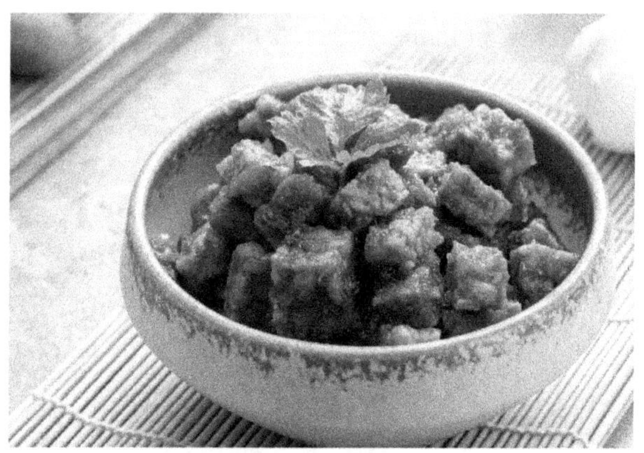

Instructions:

1. Combine soy sauce (or tamari), brown sugar (or maple syrup), sesame oil, rice vinegar, grated ginger, chopped garlic, and gochujang in a bowl.
2. Make sure the tempeh strips are properly coated before adding them to the marinade. For optimal effects, let the marinade for at least 30 minutes or overnight in the refrigerator.
3. In a skillet, preheat the heat to medium-high. Add the marinated tempeh strips and heat for 3–4 minutes on each side, or until caramelized and crispy.
4. After the tempeh is cooked, top it with chopped green onions and sesame seeds.
5. Serve hot Korean BBQ tempeh with steamed veggies and rice, or use it as a filler for wraps or sandwiches.

Mapo Tofu

Ingredients:

- 1 block (about 14 ounces) firm tofu, cubed
- 2 tablespoons vegetable oil
- 2 cloves garlic, minced
- 1 tablespoon grated ginger
- 2 green onions, thinly sliced
- 2 tablespoons fermented black beans, rinsed and chopped
- 2 tablespoons doubanjiang (spicy bean paste)
- 1 tablespoon soy sauce or tamari
- 1 teaspoon sesame oil
- 1 cup vegetable broth
- 1 teaspoon cornstarch mixed with 2 tablespoons water (for thickening)
- Cooked rice, for serving
- Sliced green onions, for garnish

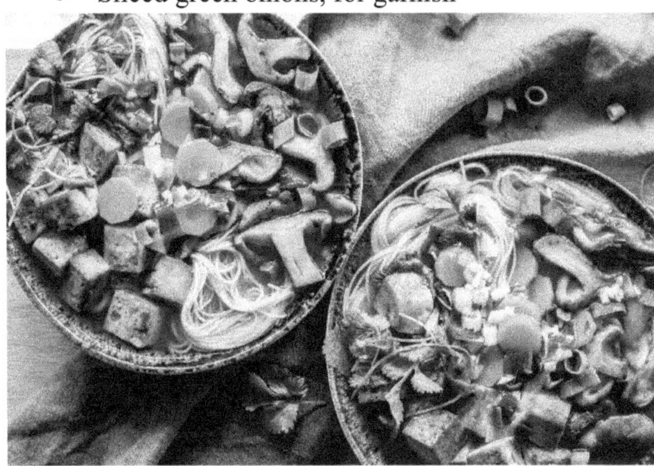

Instructions:

1. In a large skillet or wok, heat the vegetable oil over medium heat. Add the thinly sliced green onions, grated ginger, and chopped garlic. Cook for one to two minutes, or until aromatic.
2. To the skillet, add the doubanjiang and fermented black beans. Stir-fry for an additional moment.
3. When the cubed tofu is added to the skillet, gently stir it with the spices and aromatics.
4. Add the vegetable broth, sesame oil, and soy sauce (or tamari). To enable flavors to mingle, bring to a simmer and cook for five to seven minutes.
5. To thicken the sauce, stir in the cornstarch-water combination. Simmer for two to three more minutes, or until the sauce thickens and becomes glossy.
6. Taste and adjust seasoning, adding extra soy sauce as necessary.
7. Top heated Mapo tofu with cooked rice and chopped green onions as a garnish.

Teriyaki Glazed Tofu

Ingredients:

- 1 block (about 14 ounces) extra firm tofu, pressed and sliced

- 1/4 cup soy sauce or tamari
- 2 tablespoons maple syrup or brown sugar
- 1 tablespoon rice vinegar
- 1 teaspoon grated ginger
- 2 cloves garlic, minced
- 1 tablespoon cornstarch
- 2 tablespoons water
- 1 tablespoon sesame seeds
- Sliced green onions, for garnish

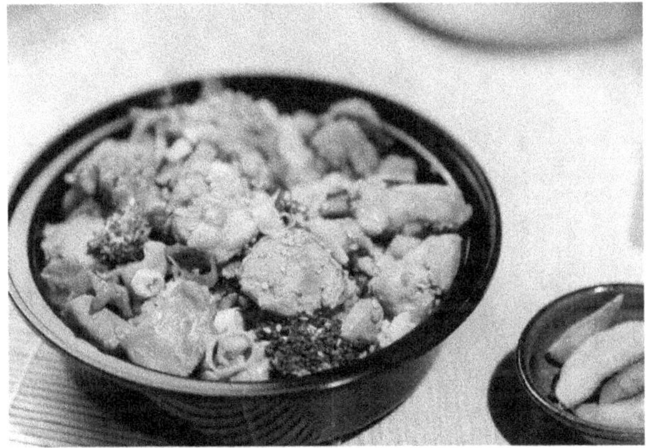

Instructions:

1. To create the teriyaki sauce, combine the soy sauce (or tamari), rice vinegar, maple syrup (or brown sugar), grated ginger, and chopped garlic in a small bowl.
2. Make a slurry out of cornstarch and water in a different bowl.
3. In a skillet, preheat to medium. Add the tofu slices and heat for 3–4 minutes on each side, or until golden brown on both sides.

4. Cover the tofu in the pan with the teriyaki sauce.
    Simmer for two to three minutes, or until the
    sauce thickens and covers the tofu.
5. Add sesame seeds to the tofu.
6. Serve hot teriyaki-glazed tofu with steamed
    veggies and rice, topped with sliced green
    onions.
7. Savor your tasty and filling plate of teriyaki
    tofu!

Curries and Stir-Fries

Thai Green Curry

Ingredients:

- 1 tablespoon vegetable oil
- 2 tablespoons Thai green curry paste
- 1 can (13.5 ounces) coconut milk
- 1 cup vegetable broth
- 1 block (about 14 ounces) tofu, cubed
- 1 cup mixed vegetables (such as bell peppers, bamboo shoots, carrots, and snap peas)
- 1 tablespoon soy sauce or tamari
- 1 tablespoon coconut sugar or brown sugar
- 1 tablespoon lime juice
- Fresh Thai basil leaves, for garnish
- Cooked jasmine rice, for serving

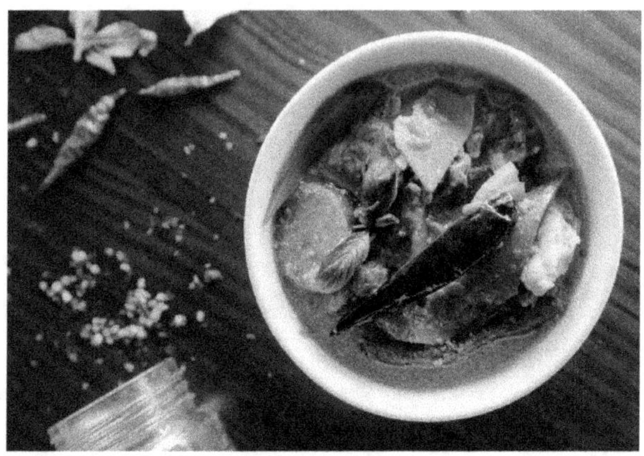

Instructions:

1. In a large skillet or wok, heat the vegetable oil over medium heat.
2. Put the paste for Thai green curry onto the pan. Stir-fry until aromatic, about one to two minutes.
3. Pour in the vegetable broth and coconut milk. Simmer after stirring to blend flavors.
4. To the skillet, add the mixed veggies and cubed tofu. Simmer for 8 to 10 minutes, or until the tofu is well cooked and the veggies are soft.
5. Add the lime juice, coconut sugar (or brown sugar), and soy sauce (or tamari).
6. To let the flavors combine, simmer for a further two to three minutes.
7. If necessary, taste and adjust the seasoning.
8. Serve hot jasmine rice with Thai green curry.
9. Before serving, garnish with fresh sprigs of Thai basil.
10. Savor your fragrant and tasty Thai green curry!

Ingredients:

- 2 medium-sized eggplants, cut into bite-sized cubes
- 2 tablespoons vegetable oil
- 3 cloves garlic, minced
- 1 tablespoon grated ginger
- 2 green onions, thinly sliced
- 2 tablespoons Szechuan peppercorns
- 1 red bell pepper, thinly sliced
- 1 yellow bell pepper, thinly sliced
- 1 tablespoon soy sauce or tamari
- 1 tablespoon rice vinegar
- 1 tablespoon maple syrup or coconut sugar
- 2 tablespoons chili garlic sauce
- Cooked rice, for serving

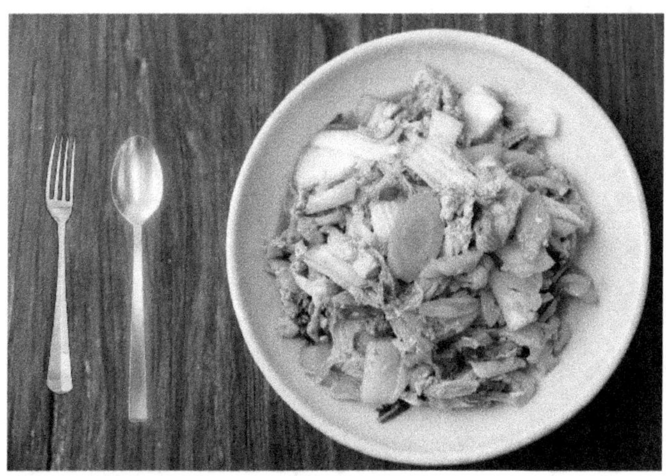

Instructions:

1. In a large skillet or wok, heat the vegetable oil over medium-high heat.
2. To the pan, add the sliced green onions, grated ginger, and chopped garlic. Sauté until aromatic, approximately 1 minute.
3. Toss in the Szechuan peppercorns and toast for an additional one to two minutes, or until fragrant.
4. To the skillet, add the cubed eggplant. Stir-fry the eggplant for 5 to 7 minutes, or until it starts to soften and get a little brown.
5. Slice the red and yellow bell peppers thinly and add them to the skillet. Stir-fry the veggies for a further three to four minutes, or until they are crisp-tender.
6. Combine rice vinegar, soy sauce (or tamari), maple syrup (or coconut sugar), and chile garlic sauce in a small bowl.

7. Over the veggies in the skillet, pour the sauce. Coat evenly by tossing, then cook for a further two to three minutes.

8. Serve hot stir-fried Szechuan eggplant over cooked rice.

Coconut Curry Vegetables

Ingredients:

- 2 tablespoons coconut oil
- 1 onion, diced
- 3 cloves garlic, minced
- 1 tablespoon grated ginger
- 2 carrots, sliced
- 1 bell pepper, sliced
- 1 zucchini, sliced
- 1 cup broccoli florets
- 1 cup cauliflower florets
- 1 can (13.5 ounces) coconut milk
- 2 tablespoons Thai red curry paste
- 1 tablespoon soy sauce or tamari
- 1 tablespoon maple syrup or coconut sugar
- Juice of 1 lime
- Salt and pepper to taste
- Fresh cilantro for garnish
- Cooked rice or noodles for serving

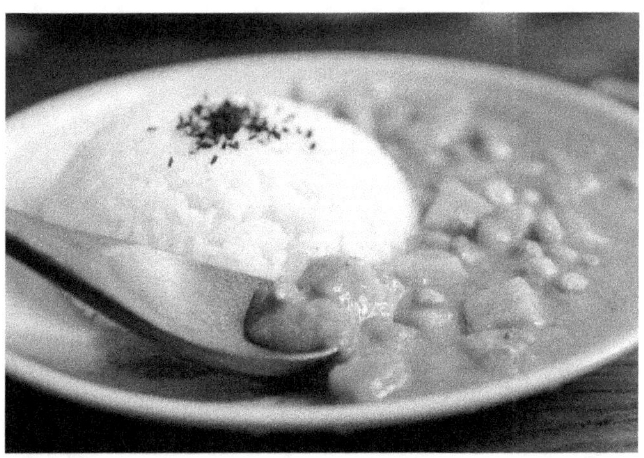

Instructions:

1. In a large skillet or wok, heat the coconut oil over medium heat.
2. To the skillet, add the chopped onion, minced garlic, and grated ginger. For about 3–4 minutes, or until the onion is transparent, sauté.
3. Carrots, bell pepper, zucchini, broccoli, and cauliflower should all be cut and added to the pan. Stir-fry the veggies for 5–6 minutes, or until they are crisp-tender.
4. Combine the coconut milk, lime juice, soy sauce (or tamari), Thai red curry paste, and maple syrup (or coconut sugar) in a small bowl.
5. Transfer the coconut milk blend onto the veggies within the skillet. Simmer after stirring to blend flavors.
6. Simmer for ten to twelve minutes, or until the sauce has somewhat thickened and the veggies are tender.

7. To taste, add salt and pepper for seasoning.
8. Serve heated veggies in a coconut curry over noodles or boiled rice.
9. Before serving, garnish with fresh cilantro.
10. Savor the flavors and creaminess of your coconut curry veggies!

Mongolian Tofu Stir-Fry

Ingredients:

- 1 block (about 14 ounces) tofu, cubed
- 2 tablespoons cornstarch
- 2 tablespoons vegetable oil
- 3 cloves garlic, minced
- 1 tablespoon grated ginger
- 2 green onions, thinly sliced
- 1/4 cup soy sauce or tamari
- 1/4 cup water
- 1/4 cup brown sugar
- 1 tablespoon rice vinegar
- 1 teaspoon sesame oil
- 1 tablespoon cornstarch mixed with 2 tablespoons water (for thickening)
- Cooked rice, for serving
- Sesame seeds, for garnish

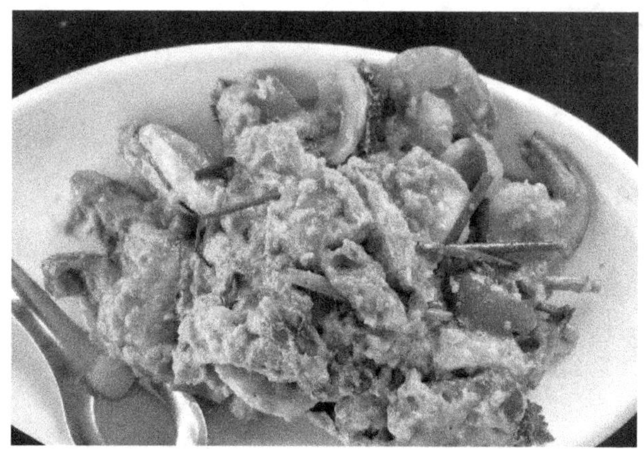

Instructions:

1. Coat the cubed tofu well with cornstarch.
2. In a large skillet or wok, heat the vegetable oil over medium-high heat.
3. Add the tofu cubes to the skillet and cook for 6 to 8 minutes, or until golden brown and crispy on both sides. Take out and put aside the tofu from the pan.
4. Add thinly sliced green onions, grated ginger, and minced garlic to the same skillet. Sauté until aromatic, about one to two minutes.
5. Mix the soy sauce (or tamari), brown sugar, rice vinegar, water, and sesame oil in a small bowl.
6. After adding the sauce to the pan, simmer it.
7. To thicken the sauce, stir in the cornstarch-water combination.
8. Return the cooked tofu to the skillet. Cook for a further two to three minutes, or until well cooked, after tossing to coat evenly in the sauce.

9. Serve hot stir-fried Mongolian tofu with cooked rice.
10. Before serving, sprinkle sesame seeds on top.
11. Savor the flavor of your stir-fried Mongolian tofu!

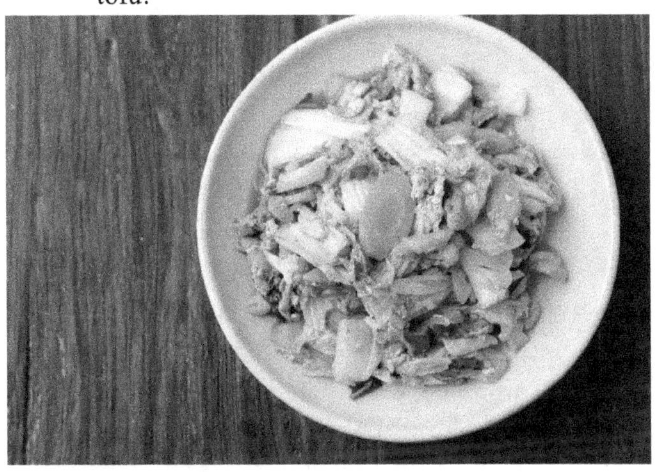

Soups and Stews

Tom Yum Soup

Ingredients:

- 4 cups vegetable broth
- 2 lemongrass stalks, bruised and chopped into 2-inch pieces
- 3 kaffir lime leaves, torn
- 3 slices galangal or ginger
- 2 Thai bird's eye chilies, sliced (adjust to taste)
- 3 cloves garlic, minced
- 1 cup mixed mushrooms (such as straw mushrooms, shiitake, or oyster mushrooms)
- 1 tomato, cut into wedges
- 1 small onion, sliced
- 2 tablespoons soy sauce or tamari
- 2 tablespoons lime juice
- 1 tablespoon coconut sugar or brown sugar
- Salt to taste
- Fresh cilantro leaves for garnish
- Thinly sliced green onions for garnish

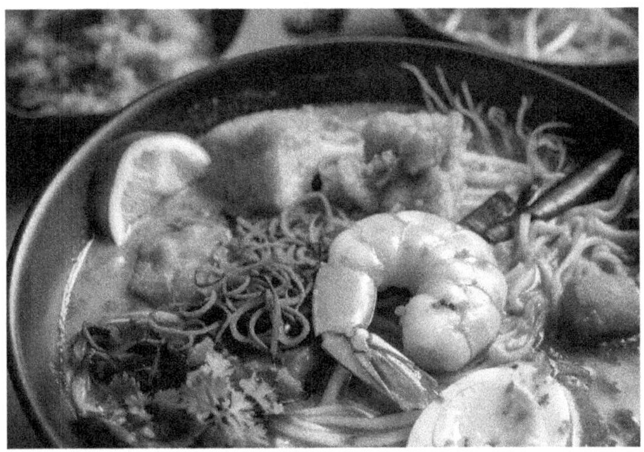

Instructions:

1. The vegetable broth should be simmered over medium heat in a large saucepan.
2. Incorporate Thai bird's eye chilies, minced garlic, galangal or ginger slices, lemongrass, and kaffir lime leaves into the mixture. Simmer for five to seven minutes to flavor the broth.
3. To the saucepan, add chopped onion, tomato wedges, and assorted mushrooms. Continue to simmer until the mushrooms are soft, about 5 to 7 minutes.
4. Add the lime juice, coconut sugar (or brown sugar), and soy sauce (or tamari). If necessary, taste and add more salt to the seasoning.
5. Before serving, remove the kaffir lime leaves and the stalks of lemongrass from the soup.
6. Spoon heated Tom Yum soup into individual bowls.
7. Add some thinly sliced green onions and fresh cilantro leaves as garnish.

8. Enjoy your tasty and fragrant Tom Yum soup
    right away!

Miso Soup with Tofu and Seaweed

Ingredients:

- 4 cups vegetable broth or dashi broth
- 3 tablespoons miso paste
- 1 block (about 14 ounces) tofu, cubed
- 2 green onions, thinly sliced
- 2 sheets nori seaweed, torn into small pieces
- 1 tablespoon soy sauce or tamari
- 1 teaspoon sesame oil
- Optional: thinly cut spinach, mushrooms, or other veggies of your choice

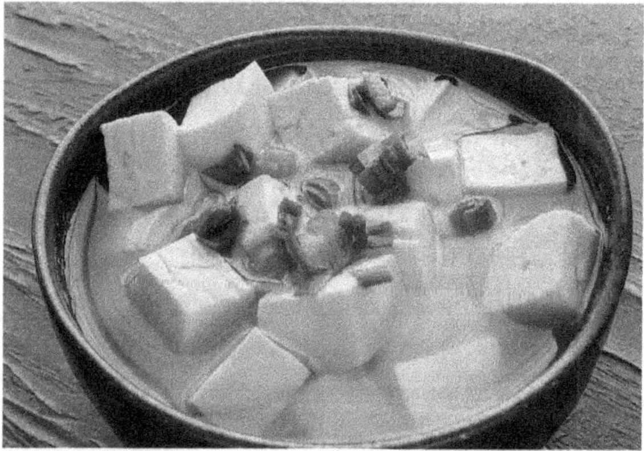

Instructions:

1. Heat a saucepan with vegetable broth or dashi broth over medium heat until it gently simmers.
2. Combine the miso paste with a ladleful of boiling soup in a small bowl and whisk until smooth.
3. Toss in the cubed tofu, chopped green onions, shredded nori seaweed, and any extra veggies.
4. Stir in soy sauce (or tamari) and miso paste combination. Simmer for two to three minutes to let the flavors combine.
5. After turning off the heat, whisk in the sesame oil.
6. If necessary, taste and adjust the seasoning.
7. Serve hot miso soup by ladling it into bowls.
8. Savor your nutritious and reassuring Miso soup with seaweed and tofu!

Spicy Korean Kimchi Stew (Kimchi Jjigae)

Ingredients:

- 2 cups kimchi, chopped
- 1/2 onion, sliced
- 2 cloves garlic, minced
- 1 tablespoon gochujang (Korean chili paste)
- 1 tablespoon gochugaru (Korean chili flakes)
- 1 tablespoon soy sauce

- 1 tablespoon sesame oil
- 4 cups vegetable broth
- 1 block (about 14 ounces) tofu, cubed
- 2 green onions, chopped
- 1 teaspoon sesame seeds for garnish (optional)

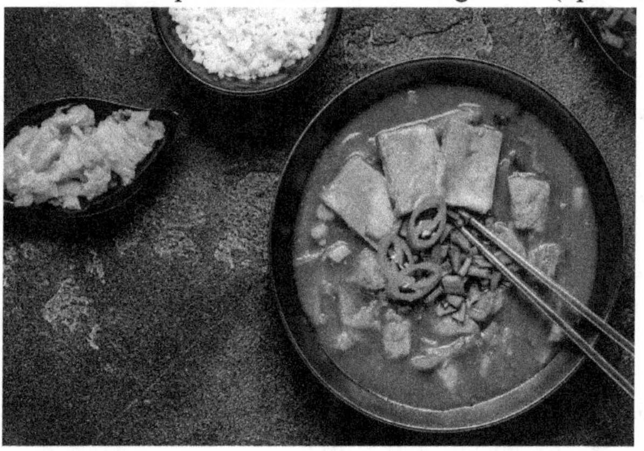

Instructions:

1. Chop the kimchi, slice the onion, mince the garlic, add the gochujang and gochugaru, soy sauce, and sesame oil to a saucepan.
2. Over medium-high heat, stir in the vegetable broth and bring to a boil.
3. To let the flavors mingle, lower the heat to low and simmer, covered, for 15 to 20 minutes.
4. Simmer the cubed tofu in the saucepan for a further five minutes.
5. If necessary, taste and adjust the seasoning.
6. Right before serving, add the chopped green onions and stir.
7. Spoon the hot Kimchi stew into individual bowls.

8. If desired, sprinkle sesame seeds on top.

9. Enjoy your spicy and soothing Korean kimchi stew hot!

Vietnamese Pho

Ingredients:

For the Broth:

- 8 cups vegetable broth
- 1 onion, halved
- 3-inch piece ginger, sliced
- 3 star anise
- 3 cloves
- 1 cinnamon stick
- 1 tablespoon soy sauce or tamari
- 1 tablespoon maple syrup or brown sugar
- Salt to taste

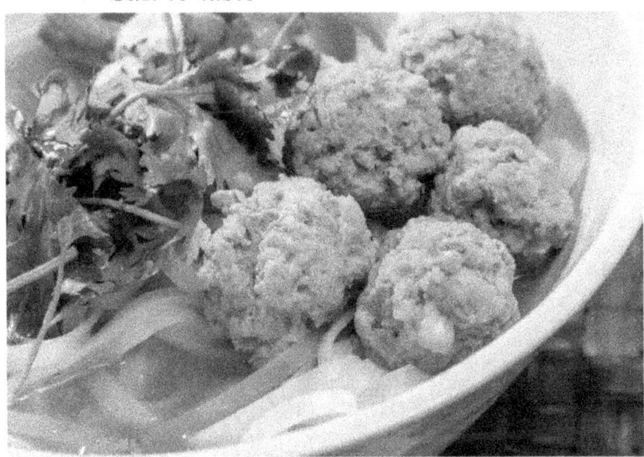

For the Soup:

- 8 ounces rice noodles
- 1 cup sliced mushrooms (shiitake, button, or cremini)
- 1 cup bean sprouts
- 1 cup thinly sliced tofu
- 2 green onions, thinly sliced
- Fresh cilantro leaves
- Lime wedges
- Thai basil leaves
- Hoisin sauce and Sriracha sauce, for serving

Instructions:

1. Vegetable broth, sliced ginger, split onion, star anise, cloves, cinnamon stick, soy sauce (or tamari), and maple syrup (or brown sugar) should all be combined in a big saucepan. To infuse flavors, bring to a boil, then lower the heat and simmer for 30 to 45 minutes.
2. Prepare the rice noodles as directed on the box while the broth simmers. After draining, set away.
3. Remove the particles from the broth by straining it through cheesecloth or a fine mesh screen. Pour the filtered soup back into the pot and add salt to taste.
4. Divide the cooked rice noodles among serving bowls to assemble the pho bowls. Add thinly sliced tofu, bean sprouts, and mushrooms over top.

5. Over the noodles and toppings in each dish,
    ladle heated broth.
6. Serve hot Vietnamese pho with fresh cilantro
    leaves, lime wedges, Thai basil leaves, and
    thinly sliced green onions as garnish.
7. For added taste, serve with Sriracha and hoisin
    sauce on the side.
8. Savor your fragrant and cozy Vietnamese pho!

Sides and Accompaniments

Jasmine Rice

Ingredients:

- 2 cups jasmine rice
- 2 1/2 cups water

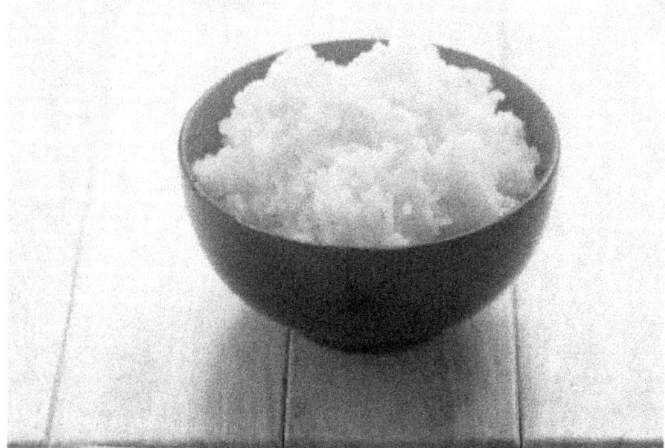

Instructions:

1. Till the water runs clear, rinse the jasmine rice under cold water. This aids in removing too much starch.
2. Rinse the jasmine rice and put it in a medium pot with water.

3. On high heat, bring the water to a boil.
4. After the saucepan reaches a boiling point, turn down the heat to low and secure the lid tightly.
5. Simmer the rice for 15 to 20 minutes, or until it is soft and all of the water has been absorbed.
6. Take the saucepan off of the burner and leave it covered for five more minutes so the rice can steam.
7. Before serving, fluff up the jasmine rice with a fork.
8. Serve the fragrant and flavorful jasmine rice as a side dish to go with your favorite Asian-inspired dishes.

Japanese Pickled Vegetables (Tsukemono)

Ingredients:

- Assorted vegetables (such as cucumbers, carrots, daikon radish, and cabbage), thinly sliced or julienned
- 1 cup rice vinegar
- 1/2 cup water
- 1/4 cup sugar
- 1 tablespoon salt

Instructions:

1. Combine rice vinegar, water, sugar, and salt in a small pot. After the sugar and salt are completely dissolved, cook over medium heat. After removing from the heat, let the brine to reach room temperature.
2. Cut the various veggies into thin slices or juice them.
3. Transfer the cut veggies to a jar or other clean glass container.
4. Make sure the veggies are completely immersed by pouring the cooled brine over them.
5. Before serving, place a lid on the jar or container and chill it for at least 24 hours.
6. Tsukemono, or pickled vegetables from Japan, may last up to two weeks in the fridge.
7. Serve as a zesty and refreshing side to your favorite Japanese dishes.

Chinese Steamed Buns (Baozi)

Ingredients:

For the Dough:

- 2 cups all-purpose flour
- 1 teaspoon active dry yeast
- 1 tablespoon sugar
- 1/2 cup warm water

For the Filling (Optional, choose your favorite):

- Minced pork or chicken with vegetables
- Tofu with vegetables
- Vegetable stir-fry
- Sweet bean paste

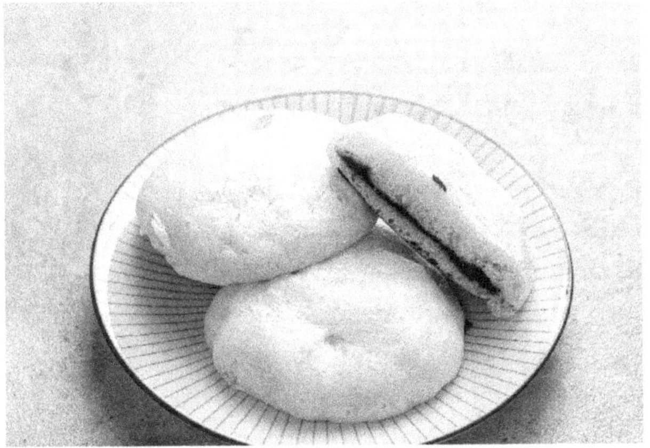

Instructions:

1. In a small bowl, combine active dry yeast, sugar, and warm water. Let it sit for about 5 minutes until frothy.
2. In a large mixing bowl, combine all-purpose flour and the yeast mixture. Mix until a dough forms.
3. Knead the dough on a floured surface for about 5-7 minutes until smooth and elastic.
4. Place the dough in a lightly oiled bowl, cover with a damp cloth, and let it rise in a warm place for about 1 hour, or until doubled in size.
5. Punch down the risen dough and divide it into small balls, about the size of a golf ball.

6.   Roll each ball into a flat circle, about 3-4 inches
     in diameter.
7.   Place a spoonful of your chosen filling in the
     center of each dough circle.
8.   Fold the edges of the dough circle up and over
     the filling, pinching them together at the top to
     seal.
9.   Place the filled buns on squares of parchment
     paper and let them rest for another 15-20
     minutes.
10. Prepare a steamer by bringing water to a boil.
11. Steam the buns in batches for about 15-20
     minutes, or until puffed and cooked through.
12. Remove the steamed buns from the steamer and
     let them cool slightly before serving.
13. Serve Chinese steamed buns (baozi) hot as a
     delicious snack or meal accompaniment.

Korean Kimchi

Ingredients:

- 1 Napa cabbage
- 1/4 cup sea salt
- 2 tablespoons sugar
- 3 cloves garlic, minced
- 1 tablespoon grated ginger
- 2 tablespoons Korean chili powder (gochugaru)
- 3 green onions, chopped

- 2 tablespoons fish sauce or soy sauce (for vegan version)
- 1 tablespoon rice vinegar

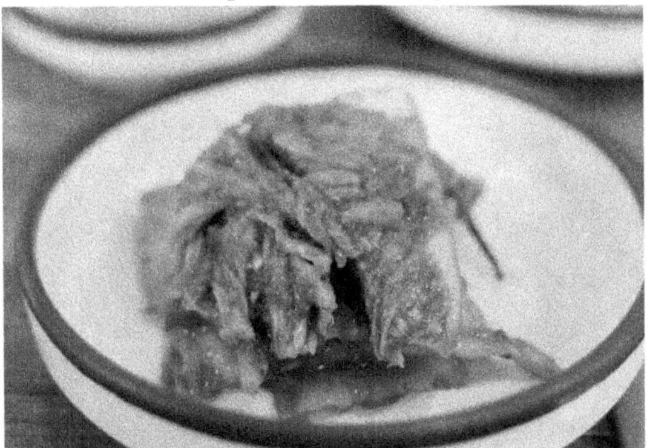

Instructions:

1. Remove the core from the Napa cabbage by cutting it into quarters lengthwise. Each quarter should be cut into 2-inch sections crosswise.
2. Eight cups of water and sea salt should be dissolved in a big dish. After adding the cabbage pieces, soak them in the salt water for two hours, turning them now and again.
3. To get rid of any extra salt, give the cabbage a good rinse in cool water. After draining, set away.
4. To prepare the kimchi paste, place chopped green onions, rice vinegar, fish sauce (or soy sauce), minced garlic, and grated ginger in a separate bowl. Add Korean chili powder.
5. Squeeze out any extra water from the cabbage pieces gently and mix them into the kimchi mixture. Evenly coat the cabbage with the paste using your hands.

6. Tightly pack the kimchi into spotless glass jars, making sure to squash any trapped air.
7. Each jar should have a gap of about 1 inch at the top before the lids are tightened.
8. After allowing the jars to ferment for one to two days at room temperature, place them in the refrigerator.
9. Before serving, let the kimchi ferment in the fridge for at least three to five days.
10. Savor Korean kimchi as a delicious and high-probiotic side dish to go with your preferred Korean cuisine or as a great addition to salads and sandwiches.

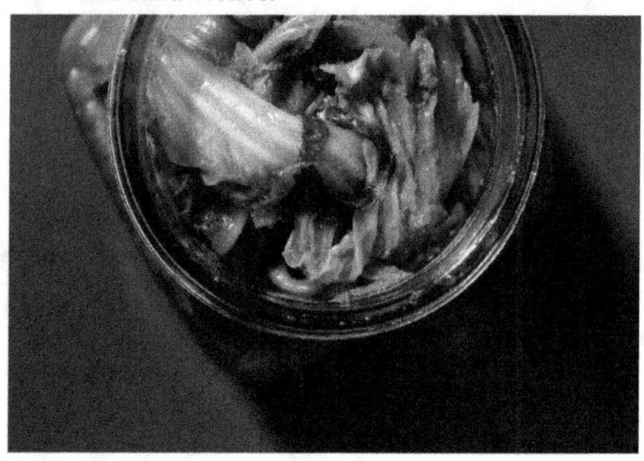

Desserts and Sweet Treats

Mango Sticky Rice

Ingredients:

- 1 cup glutinous rice (also known as sweet rice or sticky rice)
- 1 cup coconut milk
- 1/4 cup sugar
- 1/2 teaspoon salt
- 2 ripe mangoes, peeled and sliced
- Toasted sesame seeds or toasted coconut flakes, for garnish (optional)

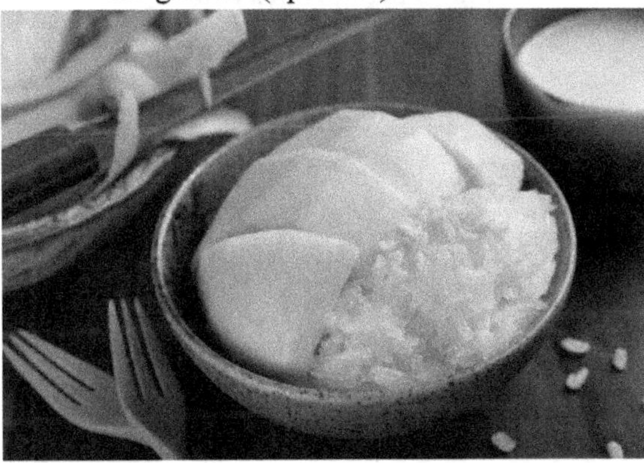

Instructions:

1. Till the water runs clear, rinse the sticky rice under cold water. Make sure to drain properly.
2. Rinse the sticky rice and put it in a saucepan with coconut milk, sugar, and salt.
3. Over medium heat, bring the mixture to a boil and then turn down the heat. Once the liquid has been absorbed and the rice is soft, cook it covered for 20 to 25 minutes.
4. Peel and slice the mangoes and set them aside while the rice cooks.
5. After the rice is done, turn off the heat and leave it alone for five minutes.
6. Spoon some cooked sticky rice onto a plate or into a dish for serving. Place mango slices next to the rice.
7. For extra taste and texture, you may optionally top the rice and mango with toasted sesame seeds or toasted coconut flakes.
8. Enjoy this delicious Thai dessert with warm or room temperature mango sticky rice!

Vegan Matcha Green Tea Ice Cream

Ingredients:

- 2 cans (13.5 oz each) full-fat coconut milk, chilled

- 1/2 cup sugar
- 2 tablespoons matcha green tea powder
- 1 teaspoon vanilla extract
- Pinch of salt

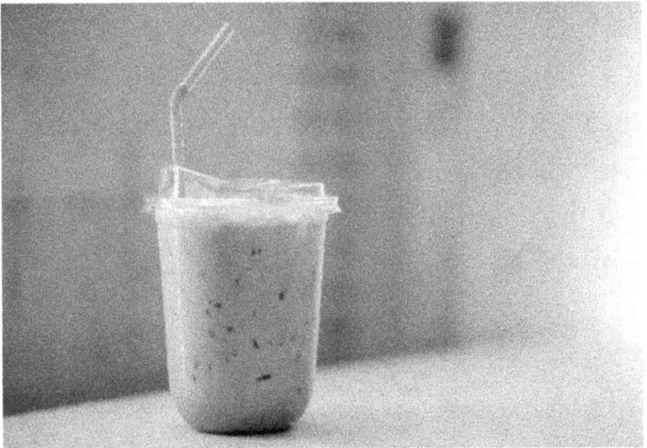

Instructions:

1. Store the coconut milk cans in the fridge for the entire night.
2. After the coconut milk cans are cold, open them and remove the thick cream that has risen to the top, discarding the liquid. The cream should be put in a mixing basin.
3. To the coconut cream, add sugar, vanilla essence, matcha green tea powder, and a little amount of salt.
4. Beat the ingredients together with a hand mixer or stand mixer until they are smooth and creamy.
5. After transferring the mixture to an ice cream machine, follow the manufacturer's directions for churning it until the consistency of soft serve is achieved.

6. To produce a creamy texture and break up ice crystals, freeze the mixture in a freezer-safe container for around 4-6 hours, stirring once every hour, if you don't have an ice cream machine.
7. When the ice cream has reached the consistency you've desired, scoop it into bowls or cones and serve right away.
8. Savor the flavor of vegan matcha green tea ice cream, which is bright and invigorating!

Coconut Tapioca Pudding

Ingredients:

- 1/2 cup small pearl tapioca
- 2 cups coconut milk
- 1/4 cup sugar
- 1/4 teaspoon salt
- 1 teaspoon vanilla extract
- Toasted coconut flakes, for garnish (optional)

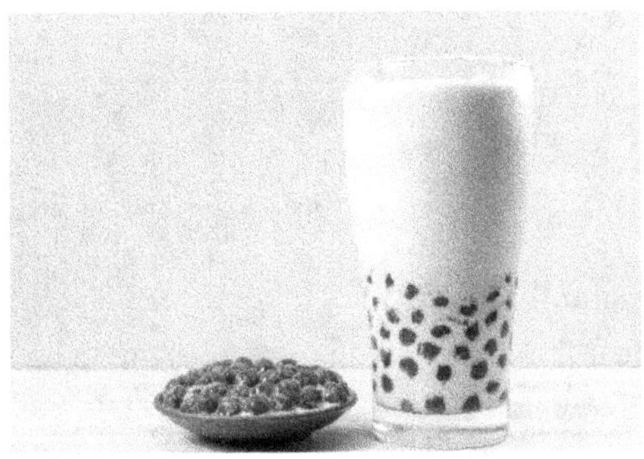

Instructions:

1. The tapioca pearls should be rinsed with cold water.
2. The washed tapioca pearls, coconut milk, sugar, and salt should all be combined in a medium pot.
3. Over medium heat, bring the mixture to a simmer, stirring often to avoid sticking.
4. After the mixture comes to a simmer, lower the heat to low and cook, stirring now and again, until the tapioca pearls are translucent and soft, 15 to 20 minutes.
5. After taking the pot off of the burner, add the vanilla essence and mix.
6. The tapioca pudding will thicken as it cools, so allow it to cool somewhat before serving.
7. If preferred, top the warm or cold coconut tapioca pudding with toasted coconut flakes.
8. Savor the smooth and cozy feel of this tapioca pudding made with coconut!

Chinese Almond Cookies

Ingredients:

- 1 cup almond flour
- 1 cup all-purpose flour
- 1/2 cup granulated sugar
- 1/2 teaspoon baking soda
- 1/4 teaspoon salt
- 1/2 cup vegetable oil
- 1 teaspoon almond extract
- Sliced almonds, for garnish (optional)

Instructions:

1. Set the oven temperature to 350°F (175°C). Grease a baking sheet gently or line it with parchment paper.
2. Almond flour, all-purpose flour, sugar, baking soda, and salt should all be combined in a mixing dish.
3. To the dry ingredients, add almond essence and vegetable oil. Stir to make a dough.
4. Form the dough into tiny balls, approximately the size of a tablespoon apiece, and arrange them on the baking sheet that has been ready. Using your palm, slightly flatten each ball.
5. As an optional garnish, place a sliced nut on top of each biscuit.

6. For 10 to 12 minutes, or until the sides are just beginning to turn golden brown, bake the cookies in the preheated oven.

7. After taking the cookies out of the oven, let them to rest for a few minutes on the baking sheet before moving them to a wire rack to finish cooling.

8. After cooling, keep the Chinese almond cookies at room temperature for up to a week by storing them in an airtight container.

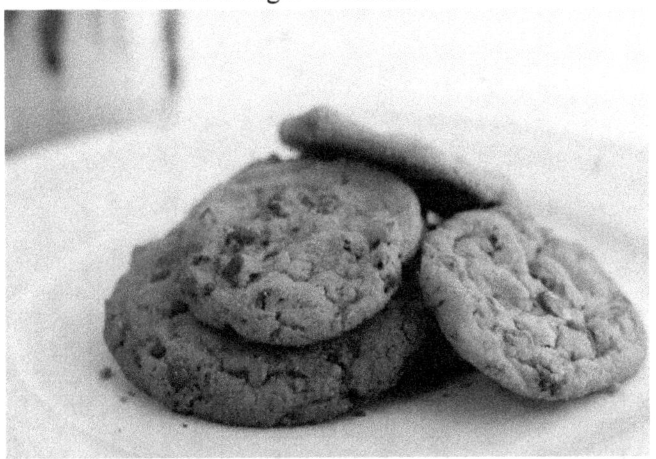

Beverages and Refreshments

Thai Iced Tea

Ingredients:

- 4 cups water
- 4 Thai tea bags (or black tea bags)
- 1/2 cup sweetened condensed milk
- Ice cubes

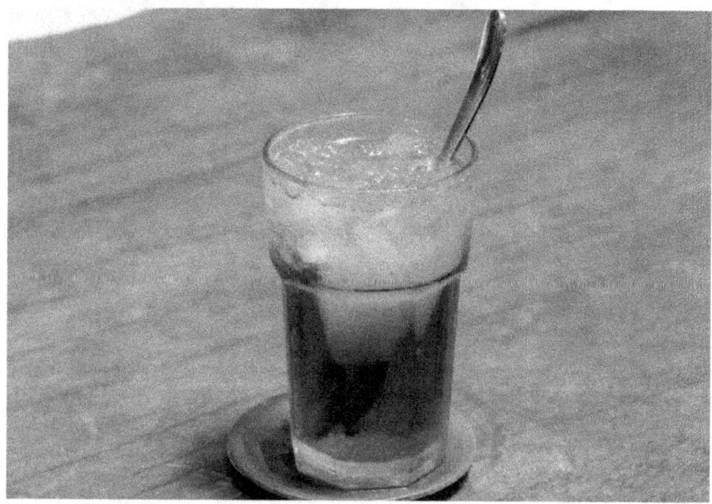

Instructions:

1. In a medium saucepan, bring 4 cups of water to a rolling boil.
2. After turning off the heat, place the Thai tea bags (or black tea bags) in the saucepan. Steep for five to seven minutes.
3. After the tea bags have steeped, remove them and carefully squeeze to release as much flavor as possible.
4. After allowing the tea to reach room temperature, place it in the refrigerator to chill for a minimum of sixty minutes.
5. When ready to serve, place ice cubes in glasses and cover the ice with the iced tea.
6. Pour a small amount of sweetened condensed milk, to taste, over the rim of each glass.
7. Mix the tea and condensed milk well by stirring.
8. If preferred, garnish with a lemon slice or a sprig of mint.
9. Savor your smooth and revitalizing Thai iced tea!

Japanese Matcha Latte

Ingredients:

- 1 teaspoon matcha green tea powder
- 2 tablespoons hot water
- 1 cup milk (dairy or plant-based)

- **1-2 teaspoons honey or sugar (optional)**

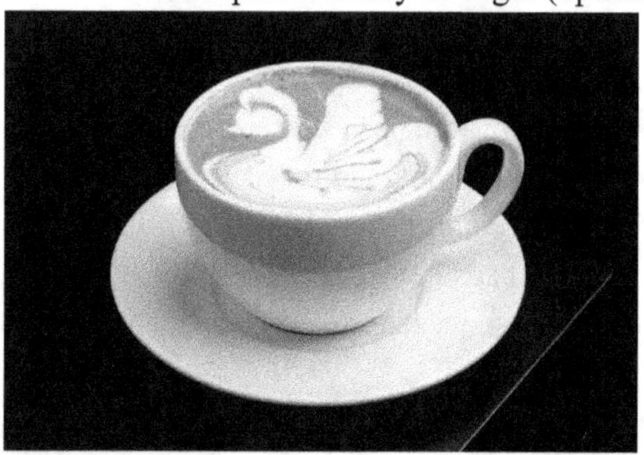

Instructions:

1. Mix matcha green tea powder and boiling water in a bowl until well combined and foamy.
2. Heat the milk in a small saucepan over medium heat until it begins to steam but does not boil.
3. Stir the sugar or honey, if using, into the heated milk until it dissolves.
4. Transfer the hot milk into a cup.
5. Pour the prepared matcha mixture slowly into the cup with the milk, and mix it in with a gentle whisk.
6. For a creamier texture, you may optionally froth the matcha latte using a portable frother.
7. Enjoy your cozy Japanese matcha latte while it's still hot!

Korean Citron Tea

Ingredients:

- 2-3 tablespoons Korean citron tea concentrate (yuzu tea)
- Hot water
- Honey, to taste (optional)

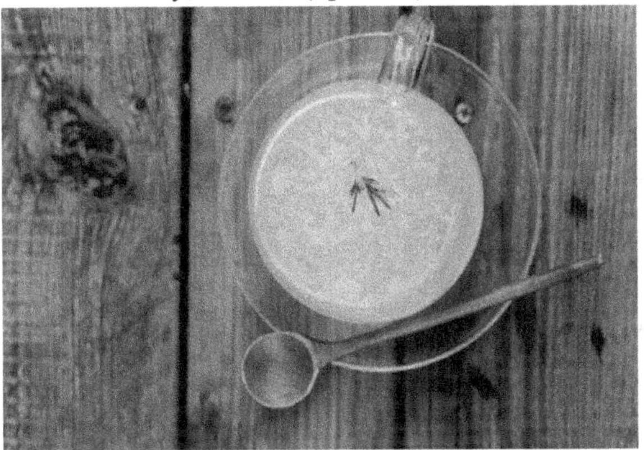

Instructions:

1. Add two to three teaspoons of concentrated Korean yuzu tea (citrus tea) to a cup.
2. Fill the mug with boiling water after adding the citron tea concentrate.
3. Make sure the hot water and concentrate are properly mixed.
4. After tasting the tea, you can alter the sweetness to your satisfaction by adding honey if desired.
5. Once the honey has completely dissolved, stir.
6. Before serving, allow the tea to cool somewhat.
7. Savor the aromatic and calming Korean citron tea as a pleasant drink or on a cold day!

Ingredients:

- 2 tablespoons finely ground Vietnamese coffee (or any dark roast coffee)
- 1/4 cup sweetened condensed milk
- Ice cubes

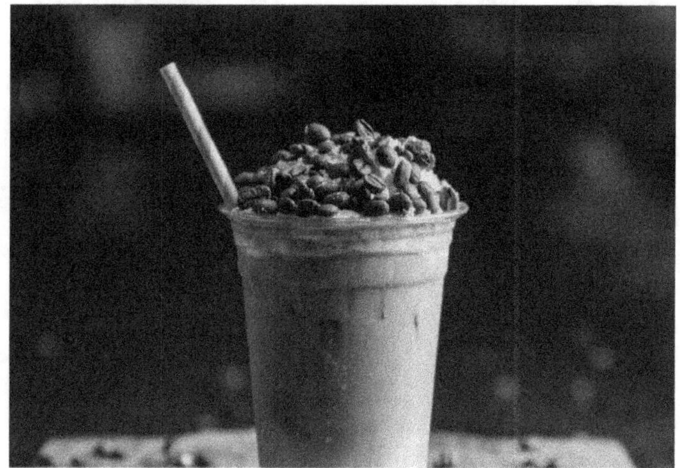

Instructions:

1. Use a drip coffee machine or a Vietnamese coffee filter to brew the finely ground coffee.
2. Pour the coffee over a glass of ice cubes while it is still hot.
3. To taste, add more or less sweetened condensed milk to the glass.
4. Make sure the coffee and condensed milk are thoroughly mixed.

5. If you would like to cool the coffee even further, add more ice cubes.

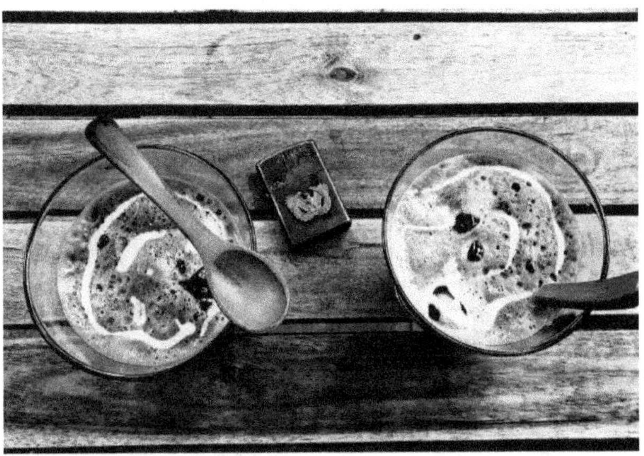

Tips for Cooking Asian Vegan Cuisine

- **Discover Common Asian Ingredients:** Become acquainted with soy sauce, coconut milk, sesame oil, miso, tofu, tempeh, seaweed, rice vinegar, and other common Asian spices and herbs. These components give your food more flavor and authenticity.

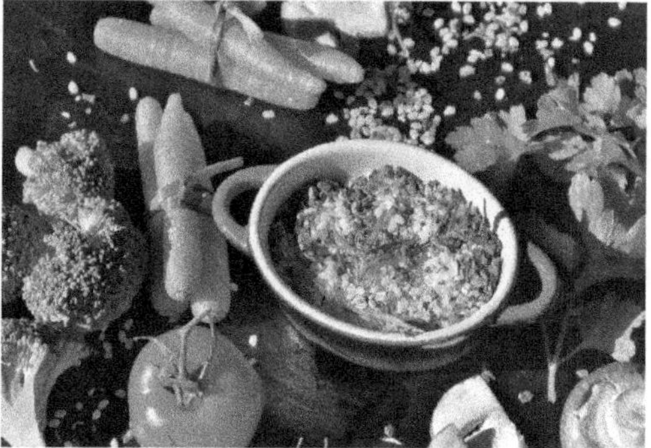

- **Try Different Plant-Based Proteins:** Tofu and tempeh are adaptable plant-based proteins that are frequently utilized in Asian cooking. To include these products into your meals, learn various culinary methods including baking, grilling, stir-frying, and marinating.

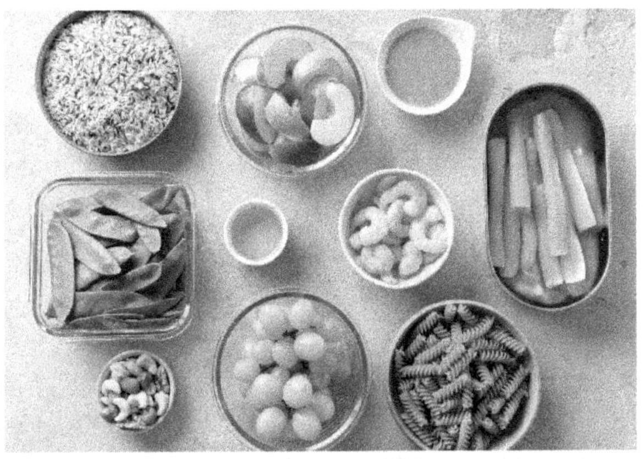

- **Master Asian Seasonings and Sauces:** Acquire the knowledge to prepare and utilize classic Asian sauces, such as sriracha, hoisin sauce, teriyaki sauce, and soy sauce. Try blending various herbs, spices, and seasonings to create distinctive taste profiles.

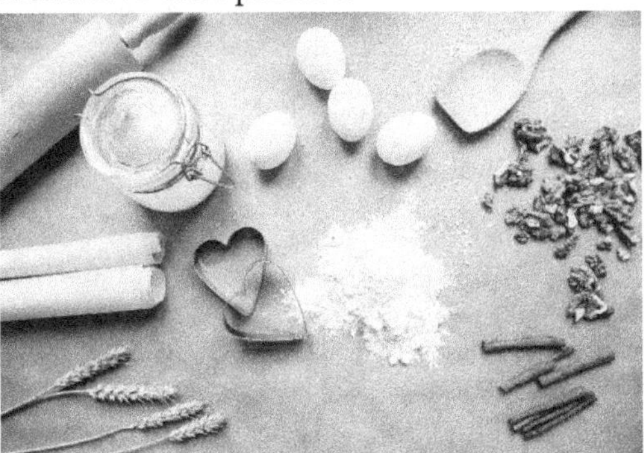

- Asian cuisine frequently combines opposing textures with a harmony of tastes, including sweet, salty, sour, and umami. Try experimenting with ingredients such as ginger, garlic, lime, and chile to make your recipes taste harmoniously balanced in terms of flavors and textures.

- **Accept Stir-Frying:** Often utilized in Asian food, stir-frying is a rapid, healthful cooking technique. For a tasty and wholesome supper, stir-fry noodles, tofu, tempeh, and veggies in a wok or big pan with flavorful sauces and spices.

- **Add Fresh Herbs and Aromatics:** Asian cuisine benefits from the vivid tastes and scents of fresh herbs such as lemongrass, Thai basil, cilantro, and mint. Aromatics, such as shallots, garlic, and ginger, are crucial for giving your meals depth of flavor.

- **Discover Asian Noodles and Rice meals:** Asian cuisine includes many different types of noodles and rice meals, including bibimbap, pad Thai, pho, sushi, and fried rice. To make a variety of tasty meals, try experimenting with different kinds of rice (jasmine rice, sushi rice, sticky rice) and noodles (rice noodles, soba noodles, udon noodles).

- **Take Your Time Choosing Plant-Based Alternatives:** Examine plant-based options including seitan, jackfruit, mushrooms, and textured vegetable protein (TVP) as alternatives to meat and fish. You may use these products to make authentic Asian cuisine without compromising on taste or texture.

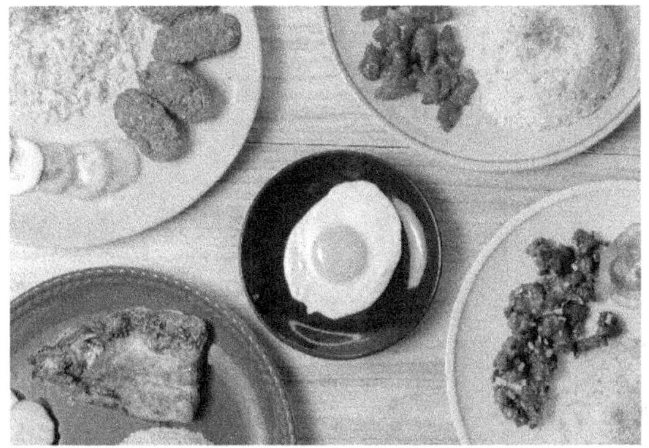

- **Learn classic culinary Methods:** Steaming, braising, pickling, and fermenting are some classic Asian culinary methods that might serve as inspiration. By using these methods, the nutritional content of plant-based products may be preserved while their natural tastes are enhanced.

- **Try New Things and Have Fun:** Don't be scared to try out new tastes, ingredients, and cooking techniques. Cooking Asian vegan food is all about having fun, being creative, and discovering new recipes to make for your family and friends.

Conclusion and Final Thoughts

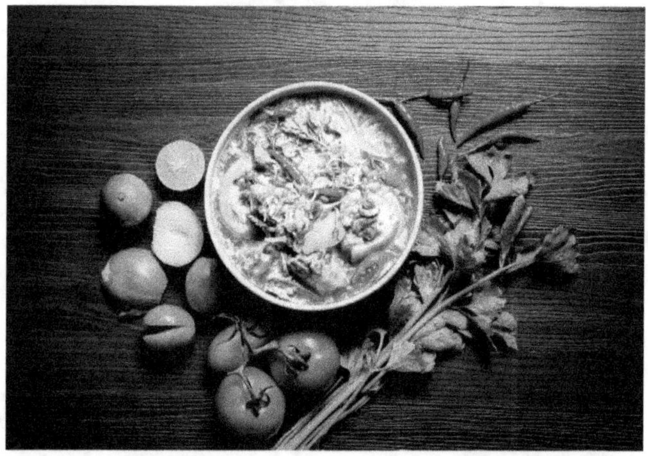

Learning about Asian vegan cooking can inspire and excite cooks of all skill levels with its diverse array of flavors, textures, and culinary traditions. We have explored the colorful and varied landscapes of Asian culinary history throughout this cookbook adventure, embracing plant-based ingredients to produce scrumptious and fulfilling recipes.

Asian vegan food honors centuries-old culinary traditions while celebrating the bounty of nature, from the comforting warmth of Korean bibimbap to the refreshing tang of Vietnamese spring rolls, and from the fragrant spices of Thai curries to the umami-rich tastes of Japanese miso soup.

Through our investigation, we have learned about the significance of using fresh, in-season ingredients, the adaptability of tofu, the artistry of stir-frying, and the delicate balance of tastes. We now understand the significance of harmony and balance in every meal as well as the complex dance of sweet, salty, sour, and spicy sensations.

As we come to the end of our culinary exploration through the pages of this Asian vegan cookbook, let's continue to cook with an adventurous, creative, and mindful mindset. I hope that these recipes will provide endless culinary adventures and strengthen our bond with the food and the civilizations that provide it.

Above all, let us keep in mind that cooking is about more than just providing for the physical needs of a family; it's also about nourishing the spirit, encouraging camaraderie, and savoring the richness of variety in our world. Whether you're preparing food for your loved ones, friends, or yourself, may every meal be an expression of compassion, love, and life.